Wall Pilates for Seniors

A Step-by-Step Unlocking Strength, Flexibility & Endurance

Willard Dean

Table of Contents

Introduction

Are you a senior looking to improve your overall fitness and well-being? If so, you're not alone. As we age, it's more important than ever to focus on building strength, improving flexibility, and enhancing balance and coordination. That's where Pilates comes in.

Here's everything you need to know about wall Pilates for seniors. Pilates is a low-impact type of exercise that prioritizes correct physical alignment, abdominal strengthening, and respiration regulation. The objective of Pilates is to strengthen the inner abdominal and back muscles that support the vertebrae while strengthening and stretching the muscles of the hips, quadriceps, and limbs. Pilates is appropriate for individuals of all ages and exercise abilities. In reality, many physical therapists use Pilates movements to help their patients recuperate from accidents. Wall Pilates is identical to conventional Pilates in that it employs deliberate, controlled exercises to tone and elongate the muscles. The distinction is that wall Pilates is practiced with the assistance of a wall (or other support). This makes it a fantastic choice for newcomers who are still acquiring the correct posture and technique.

As we grow older, it's normal to experience a decrease in muscular strength and bone integrity, leading to a whole array of problems, including an increased chance of accidents and fractures. Fortunately, Pilates is an excellent method to counteract these impacts of aging, as it concentrates on developing strength, increasing flexibility, and enhancing balance and coordination.

One of the most efficient Pilates movements for seniors is the Wall Pilates Exercise. This low-impact exercise utilizes a strong wall for support, making it a secure and approachable choice for retirees of all fitness levels.

In this book, we'll delve deep into the realm of Wall Pilates for seniors, providing step-by-step guidance to getting started with this highly effective exercise. We'll cover everything from the fundamentals of Pilates to the particular advantages of the Wall Pilates Exercise, as well as provide professional hints and guidance for getting the most out of your practice.

Whether you're a senior seeking to enhance your general fitness and well-being, or a caretaker looking for safe and effective activities for your loved one, this guide is an important reference for anyone interested in Pilates for seniors.

Throughout the book, we'll concentrate on the essential components of successful Pilates exercise, including correct breathing, posture, and alignment. We'll also examine how Pilates can help seniors develop strength, improve flexibility, and increase balance and coordination, all of which are critical for maintaining independence and quality of life as we age.

Perhaps most significantly, we'll provide a comprehensive explanation of the Wall Pilates Exercise, including step-by-step instructions and expert advice for getting the most out of each position. We'll also explore the particular advantages of this exercise, including improved equilibrium, increased flexibility, and enhanced abdominal strength.

Throughout the book, we'll highlight the significance of a secure and effective Pilates practice, providing hints and guidelines for averting damage and optimizing outcomes. We'll also address common concerns and inquiries related to Pilates for the seniors, such as how to get started with a new exercise regimen, what to do if you have a pre-existing condition, and how to adjust movements to suit your own body and abilities.

We'll also address the greater advantages of Pilates for seniors, including enhanced mental health, decreased tension and anxiety, and increased general well-being. We'll examine how Pilates can help seniors remain active and involved in their communities, and provide direction for incorporating Pilates into your daily practice.

In short, this book is a comprehensive introduction to the world of Wall Pilates for seniors, supplying everything you need to get started with this highly effective and approachable exercise. With expert direction and straightforward instructions, you'll be on your way to increased strength, flexibility, balance, and general well-being in no time.

As a Pilates instructor, I have had the privilege of working with a wide range of clients over the years, from young athletes to seniors looking to maintain their health and well-being as they age. One particular client, however, stands out in my mind as a testament to the power of Wall Pilates for seniors.

Shirley was in her early 70s when she first came to me for Pilates instruction. She had been struggling with a number of health issues, including chronic pain, limited mobility, and balance problems. Despite these challenges, Shirley was determined to stay active and maintain her independence, and she was eager to try out Pilates as a way to improve her overall health and well-being.

We started out slowly, focusing on the basics of Pilates and building up Shirley's strength and flexibility over time. I introduced her to the Wall Pilates Exercise early on, as it's a great way for seniors to build strength and improve balance without putting too much stress on the joints.

At first, Shirley struggled with the Wall Pilates Exercise, as her balance was quite poor and her muscles were weak. However, she persevered, coming to class faithfully every week and practicing at home as well. Over time, I began to see a remarkable transformation in Shirley's health and well-being.

Not only did her balance improve dramatically, but her chronic pain began to ease as well. She was able to move more freely and with less discomfort, and she began to feel a renewed sense of confidence and vitality. In addition to the physical benefits, Shirley also found that Pilates helped to reduce her stress and anxiety, providing a much-needed sense of calm and relaxation in her daily life.

As Shirley continued to practice Pilates, she became an inspiration to those around her. She would often come to class with a big smile on her face, eager to share her progress and encourage others to give Pilates a try. Her positive attitude and determination were truly infectious, and many of my other clients were inspired to take up Pilates as well.

Looking back on Shirley's journey, I'm struck by the incredible impact that Pilates can have on seniors' lives. Through consistent practice and dedication, seniors like Shirley can improve their overall health and well-being, and maintain their independence and vitality well into their golden years. I'm grateful to have had the opportunity to work with Shirley, and to witness firsthand the transformative power of Wall Pilates for seniors.

As we get older our bodies go through a number of alterations that can make commonplace activities more challenging. For seniors, in particular, there are a number of issues that can emerge, including muscular weakening, joint discomfort, poor equilibrium, and decreased flexibility.

Fortunately, Wall Pilates Exercise is an effective and approachable method for seniors to resolve these problems and enhance their general health and well-being.

One of the primary conditions that Wall Pilates Exercise can help to resolve is muscular stiffness. As we mature, we gradually lose muscular bulk and strength, which can make commonplace activities more difficult and increase the risk of accidents and fractures. Wall Pilates Exercise concentrates on developing strength and increasing muscular tone, allowing seniors to maintain their independence and reduce the risk of injury.

Another problem that Wall Pilates Exercise can help to resolve is joint discomfort and tightness. Many seniors experience rheumatism and other conditions that can make mobility unpleasant and difficult. The moderate, low-impact nature of Wall Pilates Exercise makes it a perfect choice for seniors with joint discomfort, as it can help to improve flexibility and decrease tightness without placing excessive stress on the joints.

Poor equilibrium is another prevalent problem that can influence seniors' quality of life. Falls are a significant problem for seniors, as they can lead to serious injuries and a loss of independence. Wall Pilates Exercise can help to improve balance and coordination, making seniors more steady on their feet and decreasing the risk of accidents.

Wall Pilates Exercise can help to resolve problems related to decreased flexibility and movement. As we mature, our bodies become less flexible, which can make it tougher to accomplish commonplace chores and activities. Wall Pilates Exercise can help to improve flexibility and range of motion, making it simpler for the seniors to walk comfortably and maintain an active lifestyle.

Now, let's get into the nitty-gritty of the Wall Pilate Exercise. As the name suggests, this exercise includes using a wall for support as you progress through a number of Pilates poses

Chapter 1

What is Wall Pilate?

The lengthening and strengthening advantages of conventional Pilates can be accomplished by doing movements against a wall. Wall Pilates is an excellent method to introduce newcomers to the fundamental principles of Pilates without using any apparatus.

Wall Pilates is built on the same six principles as conventional Pilates:

Concentration: Focusing your thoughts on your movements enables you to move with greater precision and control.

Control: Doing the movements carefully and with deliberate movement will help guarantee that your muscles are doing the work, rather than propulsion.

Center: Pilates movements are intended to be conducted from your center, or core. This activates your inner abdominal muscles and serves to safeguard your lower spine.

Breath: Proper breathing helps you move more effectively and also oxygenates your blood.

Precision: Each Pilates exercise is intended to be performed with a specific purpose and technique. This enables you to get the most out of each practice.

Flow: The movements are intended to flow together effortlessly and consistently.

Who is Wall Pilates For?

Wall Pilates is appropriate for individuals of all ages and exercise abilities. The activities can be adjusted to make them simpler or more challenging, so everyone can benefit from doing them. The following individuals may find wall Pilates to be particularly beneficial:

People who are new to Pilates: Wall Pilates can help you master the fundamentals of Pilates without having to use a cushion or other apparatus.

Older people who want to enhance their equilibrium and flexibility: The movements in wall Pilates can help you remain active as you mature.

People who want a low-impact workout: Since you're only using your body weight, wall Pilates is a wonderful choice for individuals who want to prevent placing too much tension on their joints.

People with restricted mobility: The movements can be done while reclining or standing, so they're perfect for people who have difficulty getting up and down from the floor.

For people who can't afford a club subscription or expensive exercise equipment: Wall Pilates is a wonderful method to get a full-body workout without breaking the budget.

What Do Beginners Need to Know?

If you're new to Pilates, there are a few things you need to know before beginning wall Pilates. Here are a few tips:

It's A Journey

Pop society would have you believe that Pilates is all about having a six-pack and appearing like Victoria's Secret model. But the reality is that Pilates is a journey, not a destination.

You will get benefits (toned musculature, enhanced balance, increased flexibility, etc.), but they will arrive gradually. So be patient and concentrate on the process, not the ultimate objective.

Start Small

When you're beginning out, some maneuvers may seem unattainable. There could be several reasons why; maybe your muscles are feeble, or your range of motion is restricted. Whatever the reason, don't attempt to thrust yourself into a situation that you're not equipped for.

Start with minor movements and build up progressively. As your strength and flexibility increase, you'll be able to do more.

Breath Work

Breath practice is an essential component of Pilates. The movements are intended to be done with steady, even breaths. This serves to oxygenate your muscles and maintains your body comfortable.

If you discover yourself retaining your breath or panting for oxygen, you're undoubtedly doing the exercise incorrectly. Take a pause and concentrate on your respiration before proceeding.

The advantages of deep breathing go beyond Pilates; it's a wonderful method to decrease tension and enhance your general health.

Core Engagement

Engaging your core is an essential component of every Pilates practice. Your core encompasses your abdominal muscles, back muscles, and pelvis.

Engaging your core helps to safeguard your lower spine and makes the movements more effective. At first, it may seem like you're using all your muscles to activate your center.

But with repetition, you'll be able to do it without thinking. One method to determine if you're activating your core correctly is to see if your midsection shifts when you breathe. If it does, you're on the correct course.

Modify the Exercises

There's no guilt in adjusting the activities to make them simpler or more challenging. In fact, it's encouraged. As you get stronger and more flexible, you can make the activities more challenging.

If an exercise is too challenging, don't be scared to ease off and do a simpler variation. The trick is to select a setting that challenges you without going excessive.

Pay Attention to Your Body

Pilates is a low-impact type of exercise, but that doesn't mean it's risk-free. It's essential to listen to your body and not press yourself too aggressively. If you experience discomfort, halt the activity and contact a doctor or physical therapist. It's also essential to consume plenty of water and limber up before doing any Pilates movements.

Get Help

As a newcomer, it's a good notion to get assistance from a qualified Pilates instructor. They can teach you the correct technique for each practice and make sure you're doing them securely.

If you can't afford individual classes, this guide and other plenty of internet materials (books, videos, etc.) can help you get started.

How Often Should You Do Wall Pilates?

There are no clear and fast guidelines, but most professionals recommend doing Pilates at least 2-3 times per week. This allows your body enough time to recuperate between exercises. If you're just beginning out, it's a good idea to take it easy and not overuse it. Once you get more comfortable with the movements, you can increase the regularity and intensity of your routines.

Will Your Body Be Sore After Wall Pilates?

It's normal to experience some muscular stiffness after doing Pilates, particularly if you're new to the exercise. This is completely typical and generally goes gone after a day or two.

If the discomfort lasts longer than a few days, or if it's accompanied by puffiness, erythema, or temperature, contact a doctor. You may have overloaded a muscle or joint, and they'll be able to offer you particular guidance on how to recuperate.

Chapter 2: Benefits of Wall Pilates for Seniors

As we age it becomes more essential than ever to remain active and preserve excellent physical health. Exercise can help seniors improve their strength, coordination, and flexibility, which can decrease the chance of accidents and injuries, as well as enhance the general quality of life. Wall Pilates is a wonderful method to accomplish all of these advantages, without placing unnecessary pressure on the body.

So, what is Wall Pilates? It's a sort of Pilates that is conducted using a wall as a support system. By using the wall as a support, seniors can participate in a low-impact exercise that is easy on the joints, yet still highly effective in developing abdominal strength, posture, and balance.

Let's take a better look at some of the advantages of Wall Pilates for seniors.

Improved Core Strength

One of the main advantages of Wall Pilates is increased abdominal strength. Core strength is important for maintaining good posture and equilibrium, and it also serves to strengthen the vertebrae and decrease the risk of back discomfort. By completing activities like wall squats and leg raises against the wall, seniors can strengthen their core muscles, which can improve their general equilibrium and mobility.

Better Posture

Another significant advantage of Wall Pilates for seniors is enhanced balance. Poor posture is a prevalent problem among seniors, and it can contribute to a plethora of health problems, including back pain, neck pain, and migraines. By performing movements like wall angels and wall slides, seniors can learn to maintain good posture and equilibrium, which can help to ameliorate these difficulties.

Increased Flexibility

Flexibility is another essential component of excellent physical health, and it becomes even more important as we mature. Regular stretching can help to increase flexibility and minimize the chance of injury. Wall Pilates involves a variety of stretching movements, such as wall stretches and wall squats, that can help seniors improve their flexibility and range of motion.

Enhanced Balance

Maintaining excellent equilibrium is important for minimizing accidents and injuries, particularly among seniors. Wall Pilates involves movements like wall lunges and wall splits that can help seniors strengthen their balance and flexibility. By performing these movements frequently, seniors can reduce their risk of accidents and enhance their general confidence and independence.

Low-Impact Workout

One of the greatest things about Wall Pilates is that it is a low-impact exercise that is gentle on the joints. For seniors who may be struggling with rheumatism or other musculoskeletal difficulties, this is particularly essential. By using the wall as a support system, seniors can participate in challenging exercises without placing unnecessary pressure on their bodies.

Variety of Exercises

Another wonderful advantage of Wall Pilates for seniors is the diversity of movements that can be performed using the wall as a support. From wall squats and wall planks to wall angels and wall stretches, there are many different movements that can be incorporated into a Wall Pilates routine. This diversity can help to keep seniors involved and motivated, while also addressing different muscle regions and increasing general physical fitness.

Mental Health Benefits

In addition to the physical advantages, Wall Pilates can also have beneficial impacts on emotional health. Regular exercise has been shown to decrease tension, anxiety, and melancholy, and can enhance general happiness and well-being. For retirees who may be struggling with loneliness or seclusion, participating in a Wall Pilates session can also provide a social release and a feeling of community.

Accessibility

Another wonderful thing about Wall Pilates is that it is approachable to people of all fitness levels and abilities. Whether you're a seasoned competitor or a newcomer who is just beginning to exercise, Wall Pilates can be customized to suit your particular requirements and objectives. Plus, since it is a low-impact exercise, it can be a wonderful choice for seniors who may be dealing with physical restrictions or persistent discomfort.

Improved Proprioception

Proprioception is your body's capacity to perceive where it is in space. This is an essential underpinning for mobility and equilibrium

Wall Pilates activities help to strengthen proprioception by challenging your equilibrium and demanding you to regulate your movements. This can contribute to enhanced equilibrium and coordination.

Reduced Stress

The advantages of Pilates go beyond the muscular. The concentration and control necessary for the activities can help cleanse your thoughts and decrease tension. Like other types of exercise, Pilates also produces neurotransmitters, which have mood-boosting benefits.

Better Sleep

The stress-reducing benefits of Pilates can also contribute to improved slumber. If you have difficulty relaxing, consider doing some wall Pilates movements before bed. You may discover that you slumber more peacefully and wake up feeling more refreshed.

Convenient and Affordable

Finally, Wall Pilates is a convenient and inexpensive exercise choice for seniors.

Since it can be conducted using just a wall and a cushion, it can simply be done at home or in a community facility. Plus, many fitness centers and clubs offer Wall Pilates sessions, which can be an inexpensive way for retirees to participate in group exercise.

Wall Pilates is a fantastic exercise choice for seniors that provides a variety of physical and emotional health advantages. By increasing abdominal strength, posture, flexibility, balance, and general physical fitness, seniors can maintain their independence, reduce their risk of accidents and injuries, and improve their overall quality of life.

Plus, with its diversity of movements, accessibility, and affordability, Wall Pilates is a wonderful choice for retirees of all fitness levels and abilities. So why not give it a shot and see the advantages for yourself?

Chapter 3: Wall Pilates Exercises for Strength and Balance

In this Chapter, I'm going to walk you through 15 types of Wall Pilates exercises that can help you improve your strength, balance, and overall physical fitness. So grab a mat, find a wall, and let's get started!

Wall Sit

The wall sit is a classic Wall Pilates exercise that targets the legs, glutes, and core muscles. To perform a wall sit, stand with your back against a wall and lower yourself down until your thighs are parallel to the ground. Hold this position for 30 seconds to 1 minute, and then stand up and repeat.

Wall Plank

The wall plank is another great exercise for targeting the core muscles, as well as the arms and shoulders.

To perform a wall plank, stand facing a wall and place your hands on the wall at shoulder height. Step back with your feet until your body is in a straight line from head to heels, and then hold this position for 30 seconds to 1 minute.

Wall Squat

The wall squat is a variation of the wall sit that targets the thighs, glutes, and core muscles. To perform a wall squat, stand with your back against a wall and lower yourself down until your thighs are parallel to the ground. From this position, lift one foot off the ground and hold for 5 to 10 seconds, and then switch sides and repeat.

Wall Push-Up

The wall push-up is a great exercise for targeting the chest, shoulders, and triceps. To perform a wall push-up, stand facing a wall and place your hands on the wall at shoulder height. Lower your body towards the wall by bending your elbows, and then push back up to the starting position.

Wall Angels

Wall angels are a great exercise for improving posture and strengthening the upper back muscles. To perform wall angels, stand with your back against a wall and raise your arms to shoulder height, with your elbows bent at 90 degrees. Slowly slide your arms up the wall, keeping your elbows bent, and then slide them back down to the starting position.

Wall Lunge

The wall lunge is a great exercise for targeting the legs and glutes. To perform a wall lunge, stand facing a wall and place one foot behind you, with your toes touching the wall. Bend your front knee and lower yourself down into a lunge position, and then push back up to the starting position.

Wall Leg Lift

The wall leg lift is a great exercise for targeting the hip flexors and core muscles. To perform a wall leg lift, lie on your back with your legs extended up the wall. Keeping your legs straight, lift one leg up towards the ceiling and hold for 5 to 10 seconds, and then switch sides and repeat.

Wall Shoulder Stretch

The wall shoulder stretch is a great exercise for improving shoulder flexibility and mobility. To perform a wall shoulder stretch, stand facing a wall and place your hands on the wall at shoulder height. Slowly walk your hands up the wall as far as you can, and then hold for 10 to 15 seconds.

Wall Tricep Stretch

The wall tricep stretch is a great exercise for improving arm and shoulder flexibility. To perform a wall tricep stretch, stand facing a wall and place one hand on the wall at shoulder height.

Rotate your body away from the wall, stretching your arm across your chest, and then hold for 10 to 15 seconds. Switch sides and repeat.

Wall Calf Stretch

The wall calf stretch is a great exercise for improving lower leg flexibility and reducing the risk of calf strains. To perform a wall calf stretch, stand facing a wall and place one foot behind you, with your heel on the ground and your toes touching the wall. Lean into the wall, keeping your back leg straight, until you feel a stretch in your calf. Hold for 10 to 15 seconds, and then switch sides and repeat.

Wall Crunch

The wall crunch is a great exercise for targeting the abdominal muscles. To perform a wall crunch, lie on your back with your feet on the wall and your knees bent at a 90-degree angle. Place your hands behind your head, and then lift your shoulders off the ground, crunching your abs. Lower yourself back to your starting position and repeat.

Wall Reverse Plank

The wall reverse plank is a great exercise for targeting the back, glutes, and hamstrings. To perform a wall reverse plank, sit on the ground with your back against a wall and your legs extended in front of you. Place your hands on the ground behind you, with your fingers pointing towards the wall. Lift your hips off the ground, creating a straight line from your shoulders to your heels, and hold for 30 seconds to 1 minute.

Wall Leg Press

The wall leg press is a great exercise for targeting the quads and glutes. To perform a wall leg press, stand facing a wall and place your hands on the wall at shoulder height. Lift one leg off the ground and press it back into the wall, squeezing your glutes and quads. Lower your leg back down to the starting position, and then repeat on the other side.

Wall Hamstring Curl

The wall hamstring curl is a great exercise for targeting the hamstrings and glutes. To perform a wall hamstring curl, lie on your back with your feet on the wall and your knees bent at a 90-degree angle. Lift your hips off the ground, creating a straight line from your shoulders to your knees, and then curl your heels towards your glutes. Lower your heels back down to the starting position, and then repeat.

Wall Knee Raise

The wall knee raise is a great exercise for targeting the hip flexors and lower abs. To perform a wall knee raise, stand facing a wall and place your hands on the wall at shoulder height. Lift one knee up towards your chest, squeezing your lower abs, and then lower it back down to the starting position. Repeat on the other side.

There you have it, 15 types of Wall Pilates exercises that can help improve your strength, balance, and overall physical fitness. Remember to always listen to your body and start slowly if you're new to these exercises. As always, I'm here to support you on your fitness journey, so let's get moving!

Chapter 4: Wall Pilates Exercises for Flexibility and Mobility

Absolutely, let's dive into different types of Wall Pilates exercises for flexibility and mobility!

Wall Chest Stretch

The wall chest stretch is a great exercise for opening up the chest and shoulders. To perform a wall chest stretch, stand facing a wall with your arms at shoulder height and your palms against the wall. Slowly lean forward, feeling a stretch in your chest and shoulders. Hold for about ten to fifteen seconds, and then release.

Wall Shoulder Stretch

The wall shoulder stretch is a great exercise for releasing tension in the shoulders and upper back. To perform a wall shoulder stretch, stand facing a wall and place your hands on the wall at shoulder height. Slowly walk your hands down the wall, keeping your arms straight, until you feel a stretch in your shoulders and upper back.

Hold for about ten to fifteen seconds, and then release.

Wall Spine Stretch

The wall spine stretch is a great exercise for improving spinal mobility. To perform a wall spine stretch, stand facing a wall and place your hands on the wall at shoulder height.

Slowly walk your hands up the wall, arching your back, until you feel a stretch in your spine. Hold for about ten to fifteen seconds, and then release.

Wall Hip Stretch

The wall hip stretch is a great exercise for opening up the hips and improving hip mobility. To perform a wall hip stretch, stand facing a wall and place your hands on the wall at hip height. Place one foot on the wall, with your knee bent at a 90-degree angle. Slowly lean forward, feeling a stretch in your hip. Hold for 10 to 15 seconds, and then switch sides.

Wall Forward Fold

The wall forward fold is a great exercise for stretching the hamstrings and lower back. To perform a wall forward fold, stand facing a wall and place your hands on the wall at shoulder height. Slowly walk your feet back, keeping your hands on the wall, until your body forms a straight line from your hands to your heels. Relax your head and neck, and hold for 10 to 15 seconds.

Wall Lunge

The wall lunge is a great exercise for stretching the hip flexors and improving hip mobility. To perform a wall lunge, stand facing a wall and place your hands on the wall at shoulder height. Take a large step back with one foot, keeping your back leg straight and your front knee bent at a 90-degree angle. Lean into the wall, feeling a stretch in your hip flexors. Hold for 10 to 15 seconds, and then switch sides.

Wall Hamstring Stretch

The wall hamstring stretch is a great exercise for stretching the hamstrings and improving flexibility. To perform a wall hamstring stretch, lie on your back with your feet on the wall and your legs extended straight up the wall. Slowly walk your hands up your legs towards your feet, feeling a stretch in your hamstrings. Hold for about ten to fifteen seconds, and then release.

Wall Figure 4 Stretch

The wall figure 4 stretch is a great exercise for stretching the glutes and hips. To perform a wall figure 4 stretch, stand facing a wall and place your hands on the wall at shoulder height. Cross one ankle over the opposite knee, creating a figure 4 shape with your legs. Slowly lean into the wall, feeling a stretch in your glutes and hips. Hold for 10 to 15 seconds, and then switch sides.

Wall Quad Stretch

The wall quad stretch is a great exercise for stretching the quads and improving mobility. To perform a wall quad stretch, stand facing a wall and place your hands on the wall at shoulder height. Lift one foot off the ground and bend your knee, bringing your heel towards your glutes. Grasp your ankle with your hand and gently pull your foot towards your glutes until you feel a stretch in your quad. Hold for 10 to 15 seconds, and then switch sides.

Wall Calf Stretch

The wall calf stretch is a great exercise for stretching the calves and improving ankle mobility. To perform a wall calf stretch, stand facing a wall and place your hands on the wall at shoulder height. Step one foot back, keeping your heel on the ground, and lean into the wall, feeling a stretch in your calf. Hold for 10 to 15 seconds, and then switch sides.

Wall Wrist Stretch

The wall wrist stretch is a great exercise for stretching the wrists and improving wrist mobility. To perform a wall wrist stretch, stand facing a wall and place your palms on the wall at shoulder height, with your fingers pointing towards the ceiling. Slowly lean forward, feeling a stretch in your wrists. Hold for about ten to fifteen seconds, and then release.

Wall Ankle Stretch

The wall ankle stretch is a great exercise for improving ankle mobility. To perform a wall ankle stretch, sit on the floor facing a wall with your legs straight out in front of you. Place one foot against the wall, with your toes pointing towards the ceiling. Slowly lean forward, feeling a stretch in your ankle. Hold for 10 to 15 seconds, and then switch sides.

Wall Neck Stretch

The wall neck stretch is a great exercise for releasing tension in the neck and improving neck mobility. To perform a wall neck stretch, stand facing a wall and place your hands on the wall at shoulder height. Slowly tuck your chin towards your chest, feeling a stretch in the back of your neck. Hold for about ten to fifteen seconds, and then release.

Wall Upper Back Stretch

The wall upper back stretch is a great exercise for releasing tension in the upper back and improving upper back mobility. To perform a wall upper back stretch, stand facing a wall and place your hands on the wall at shoulder height. Walk your hands down the wall, keeping your arms straight, until you feel a stretch in your upper back. Hold for about ten to fifteen seconds, and then release.

Wall Quad Release

The wall quad release is a great exercise for releasing tension in the quads and improving mobility. To perform a wall quad release, stand facing a wall and place your hands on the wall at shoulder height. Take a large step back with one foot, keeping your back leg straight and your front knee bent at a 90-degree angle. Slowly release your quadricep muscle, allowing your knee to bend and your foot to move towards your glutes. Hold for 10 to 15 seconds, and then switch sides.

Incorporating these 15 types of Wall Pilates exercises into your workout routine can greatly improve your flexibility and mobility. Remember to listen to your body and go at your own pace, gradually increasing the intensity and duration of each exercise as you progress. With consistent practice, you'll notice improvements in your flexibility, mobility, and overall well-being.

Chapter 5: Wall Pilates Exercises for Posture and Core Strength

Wall Sit-Ups

Wall sit-ups are a great exercise for building core strength and improving posture. To perform a wall sit-up, lie on your back with your feet flat against the wall and your knees bent. Place your hands behind your head and engage your core muscles as you lift your head and shoulders off the ground. Lower back down and repeat for ten to twelve reps.

Wall Planks

Wall planks are a great exercise for building core strength and improving posture. To perform a wall plank, stand facing a wall and place your hands on the wall at shoulder height. Step back with your feet until your body forms a straight line from head to heels. Hold for 30 to 60 seconds, engaging your core muscles throughout the exercise.

Wall Crunches

Wall crunches are a great exercise for building core strength and improving posture. To perform a wall crunch, stand facing a wall and place your hands on the wall at shoulder height. Lift one knee towards your chest and bring your opposite elbow towards your knee, twisting your torso to engage your oblique muscles. Repeat for ten to twelve reps on each side.

Wall Bridges

Wall bridges are a great exercise for building core strength and improving posture. To perform a wall bridge, lie on your back with your feet flat against the wall and your knees bent. Place your arms by your sides and engage your glutes and core muscles as you lift your hips off the ground. Lower back down and repeat for ten to twelve reps.

Wall Side Planks

Wall side planks are a great exercise for building core strength and improving posture. To perform a wall side plank, stand facing a wall and place one hand on the wall at shoulder height. Step your feet out to the side and engage your core muscles as you lift your hips off the ground, forming a straight line from head to heels. Hold for thirty to sixty seconds on each side.

Wall Mountain Climbers

Wall mountain climbers are a great exercise for building core strength and improving posture. To perform a wall mountain climber, stand facing a wall and place your hands on the wall at shoulder height. Bring one knee towards your chest and then switch legs in a running motion, engaging your core muscles throughout the exercise. Repeat for ten to twelve reps on each side.

Wall Knee Tucks

Wall knee tucks are a great exercise for building core strength and improving posture. To perform a wall knee tuck, stand facing a wall and place your hands on the wall at shoulder height. Bring one knee towards your chest and then extend your leg straight out in front of you, engaging your core muscles throughout the exercise. Repeat for ten to twelve reps on each side.

Wall Dead Bugs

Wall dead bugs are a great exercise for building core strength and improving posture. To perform a wall dead bug, lie on your back with your feet flat against the wall and your knees bent. Raise your arms and legs towards the ceiling and engage your core muscles as you lower one arm and the opposite leg towards the ground. Alternate sides for ten to twelve reps.

Wall V-Ups

Wall V-Ups are a great exercise for building core strength and improving posture. To perform a wall V-Up, lie on your back with your feet flat against the wall and your arms extended towards the ceiling. Engage your core muscles as you lift your upper body and legs towards the ceiling, forming a V shape with your body. Lower back down and repeat for ten to twelve reps.

Wall Bird Dogs

Wall bird dogs are a great exercise for building core strength and improving posture. To perform a wall bird dog, stand facing a wall and place your hands on the wall at shoulder height. Extend one leg straight back and the opposite arm straight forward, engaging your core muscles to maintain balance. Switch sides and repeat for ten to twelve reps on each side.

Wall Knee Raises

Wall knee raises are a great exercise for building core strength and improving posture. To perform a wall knee raise, stand facing a wall and place your hands on the wall at shoulder height. Lift one knee towards your chest, engaging your core muscles throughout the exercise. Lower back down and repeat for ten to twelve reps on each side.

Wall Leg Lowers

Wall leg lowers are a great exercise for building core strength and improving posture. To perform a wall leg lower, lie on your back with your feet flat against the wall and your knees bent. Engage your core muscles as you lower one leg towards the ground, keeping the other leg bent against the wall. Alternate sides for ten to twelve reps.

Wall Superman

Wall superman is a great exercise for building core strength and improving posture. To perform a wall superman, stand facing a wall and place your hands on the wall at shoulder height. Lift both legs off the ground and extend your arms straight out in front of you, engaging your core muscles to maintain balance. Hold for thirty to sixty seconds.

Wall Knee Hugs

Wall knee hugs are a great exercise for building core strength and improving posture. To perform a wall knee hug, stand facing a wall and place your hands on the wall at shoulder height. Bring one knee towards your chest and hug it in towards your body, engaging your core muscles throughout the exercise. Repeat for ten to twelve reps on each side.

Wall Twist

Wall twist is a great exercise for building core strength and improving posture. To perform a wall twist, stand facing a wall and place your hands on the wall at shoulder height. Twist your torso to one side, bringing your opposite knee towards your chest, engaging your oblique muscles. Repeat for ten to twelve reps on each side.

Incorporating Wall Pilates exercises into your fitness routine can help improve your posture and core strength. Remember to engage your core muscles throughout each exercise to maximize the benefits. Start with a few reps of each exercise and gradually increase as you become more comfortable and confident.

Chapter 6: Wall Pilates Exercises for Proper Breathing Techniques

Breathing is an important aspect of Pilates, and incorporating proper breathing techniques can improve the effectiveness of your workout.

Wall Chest Expansion

Wall chest expansion is a great exercise to help open up your chest and improve your breathing. Stand facing a wall with your arms raised and hands on the wall at shoulder height. Take a deep breath in, and as you exhale, push your hands into the wall and round your spine. Inhale to return to the starting position and repeat for 10 to 12 reps.

Wall Roll-Down

Wall roll-down is a great exercise to help improve your breathing and spine mobility. Face a wall with your feet hip-width apart and your hands on the wall at shoulder height. Exhale as you roll your spine down towards the floor, keeping your knees bent. Inhale to return to the starting position and repeat for 10 to 12 reps.

Wall Squat

Wall squat is a great exercise to help improve your breathing and leg strength. Face a wall with your feet hip-width apart and your hands on the wall at shoulder height. Squat down as low as you can, keeping your back straight and your chest lifted. Exhale as you drop and inhale as you rise.. Repeat for 10 to 12 reps.

Wall Push-Up

Wall push-up is a great exercise to help improve your breathing and upper body strength. Face a wall and place your hands at shoulder height. Inhale as you bend your elbows and lower your chest towards the wall. Exhale as you push back up. Repeat for 10 to 12 reps.

Wall Arm Circles

Wall arm circles are a great exercise to help improve your breathing and shoulder mobility. Face a wall and place your hands at shoulder height. Take a deep breath in, and as you exhale, make small circles with your arms. Inhale to switch directions and repeat for 10 to 12 reps.

Wall Leg Lifts

Wall leg lifts are a great exercise to help improve your breathing and leg strength. Face a wall and place your hands at shoulder height. Lift one leg straight out to the side, keeping your hips and shoulders facing forward. Inhale while lifting and exhale when lowering. Repeat for ten to twelve reps.

Wall Arm Reaches

Wall arm reaches are a great exercise to help improve your breathing and upper body strength. Face a wall and place your hands at shoulder height. Reach one arm up towards the ceiling, keeping your hips and shoulders facing forward. Inhale as you reach up, and exhale as you lower. Repeat for ten to twelve reps on each side.

Wall Lunge

Wall lunge is a great exercise to help improve your breathing and leg strength. Face a wall and place your hands at shoulder height on it. Step one foot back into a lunge position, keeping your front knee over your ankle. Inhale as you drop and exhale as you raise. Repeat for ten to twelve reps on each side.

Wall Plank

Wall plank is a great exercise to help improve your breathing and core strength. Face a wall and place your hands on the wall at shoulder height. Walk your feet back until your body is in a straight line from your head to your heels. Inhale as you hold the position, and exhale as you release. Hold for 30 to 60 seconds.

Wall Calf Raises

Wall calf raises are a great exercise to help improve your breathing and calf strength. Face a wall with your hands on the wall at shoulder height. Raise up onto your toes, inhaling as you lift, and exhale as you lower back down. Repeat for 10 to 12 reps.

Wall Leg Extension

Wall leg extension is a great exercise to help improve your breathing and leg strength. Face a wall with your hands on the wall at shoulder height. Lift one leg straight back behind you, keeping your hips and shoulders facing forward. Inhale while lifting and exhale when lowering. Repeat for ten to twelve reps on each side.

Wall Triceps Push-Up

Wall triceps push-up is a great exercise to help improve your breathing and arm strength. Stand facing a wall with your hands on the wall at shoulder height and slightly wider than shoulder-width apart. Inhale as you bend your elbows and lower your chest towards the wall, keeping your elbows close to your body. Exhale as you push back up. Repeat for 10 to 12 reps.

Wall Side Bend

Wall side bend is a great exercise to help improve your breathing and side body strength. Stand facing a wall with one hand on the wall at shoulder height. Reach your other arm up towards the ceiling, inhaling as you lengthen your side body. Exhale as you lower back down. Repeat for ten to twelve reps on each side.

Wall Knee Lifts

Wall knee lifts are a great exercise to help improve your breathing and core strength. Face a wall with your hands on the wall at shoulder height. Lift one knee up towards your chest, inhaling as you lift, and exhale as you lower back down. Repeat for ten to twelve reps on each side.

Wall Side Plank

Wall side plank is a great exercise to help improve your breathing and side body strength. Face a wall and place your forearm on the wall at shoulder height. Walk your feet away from the wall and lift your hips up towards the ceiling, creating a straight line from your head to your heels. Inhale as you hold the position, and exhale as you release. Hold for thirty to sixty seconds on each side.

Incorporating these 15 types of Wall Pilates exercises for proper breathing techniques into your Pilates routine can help you improve your breathing, enhance your overall Pilates practice, and provide additional health benefits.

Chapter 7: Safety Considerations for Wall Pilates Exercises

Wall Pilates exercises are a great way to improve your strength, flexibility, balance, and overall health. However, as with any form of exercise, there are certain safety considerations that need to be taken into account to ensure that you perform the exercises safely and avoid injury.

In this chapter, we will discuss some of the key safety considerations for Wall Pilates exercises.

Warm-Up

Before you begin any Wall Pilates exercise, it is essential to warm up your body. This will help to increase blood flow to your muscles, prepare your body for exercise, and reduce the risk of injury.

A good warm-up for Wall Pilates exercises could include walking, gentle stretching, or a few minutes of low-intensity cardio, such as jumping jacks or marching on the spot.

Proper Alignment

Proper alignment is essential when performing Wall Pilates exercises. Incorrect alignment can lead to poor form, which can increase the risk of injury and reduce the effectiveness of the exercise.

To ensure proper alignment, make sure that your shoulders are stacked over your hips, and your hips are stacked over your ankles. Keep your spine in a neutral position, with your head in line with your spine. Also, be sure to engage your core muscles throughout the exercises to support your back and protect your spine.

Controlled Movements

Wall Pilates exercises are all about controlled movements. This means that you should move slowly and deliberately through each exercise, focusing on proper form and alignment.

Avoid sudden, jerky movements, as these can increase the risk of injury. Instead, move with intention, and focus on the quality of the movement rather than the quantity.

Proper Breathing

Proper breathing is crucial when performing Wall Pilates exercises. Focusing on your breath can help to improve your concentration, reduce stress, and provide a deeper connection to your body.

In Wall Pilates, you should inhale through your nose and exhale through your mouth, focusing on deep, diaphragmatic breathing. Try to coordinate your breath with the movements, inhaling as you prepare for the movement and exhaling as you perform it.

Modifications

Modifications can be an excellent way to tailor Wall Pilates exercises to your individual needs. Modifications can be made to make an exercise easier or more challenging, depending on your level of fitness.

If you are new to Wall Pilates, start with the beginner-level exercises and gradually work your way up to more challenging exercises. If you have any injuries or limitations, speak to your Pilates instructor about modifications that can be made to accommodate your needs.

Hydration

Staying hydrated is essential when performing Wall Pilates exercises. Drink plenty of water before, during, and after your workout to help keep your body hydrated and maintain your energy levels.

Rest and Recovery

Rest and recovery are just as important as exercise when it comes to Wall Pilates. Make sure to give your body plenty of time to rest and recover between workouts to avoid overtraining and reduce the risk of injury.

Progression

Progression is an essential part of any exercise program, including Wall Pilates. As you become stronger and more confident in your Wall Pilates practice, gradually increase the intensity or duration of your workouts to continue to challenge your body and improve your fitness level.

Proper Equipment

Using proper equipment is essential when performing Wall Pilates exercises. Make sure to use a sturdy wall or Pilates wall unit that can support your weight and provide stability during the exercises.

Also, use proper footwear with good grip and support to help prevent slips and falls. Avoid using socks or bare feet, as these can be slippery on some surfaces.

Seek Professional Guidance

Finally, it is essential to seek professional guidance when performing Wall Pilates exercises, especially if you are new to the practice or have any injuries or limitations.

Working with a certified Pilates instructor can help you learn proper form and technique, provide modifications to accommodate your individual needs, and ensure that you are performing the exercises safely and effectively.

Conclusion

In conclusion, Wall Pilates exercises can be an excellent way for seniors to improve their overall health and fitness. These exercises are low-impact, gentle on the joints, and can be easily modified to accommodate individual needs and limitations.

Wall Pilates exercises can improve strength, balance, flexibility, mobility, posture, and proper breathing techniques. These exercises can also help seniors maintain independence, reduce the risk of falls, and improve overall quality of life.

It is important for seniors to take certain safety considerations into account when performing Wall Pilates exercises. It is recommended to warm up before each exercise, focus on proper alignment and controlled movements, and use proper breathing techniques. Modifications should be made to tailor the exercises to individual needs, and seniors should stay hydrated throughout their workout.

Rest and recovery are just as important as exercise when it comes to Wall Pilates, so seniors should give their bodies plenty of time to rest and recover between workouts. Seeking professional guidance from a certified Pilates instructor can also ensure that exercises are performed safely and effectively.

Incorporating Wall Pilates exercises into a senior's fitness routine can have a significant impact on their overall health and well-being. By taking the time to learn and perform these exercises safely and effectively, seniors can enjoy all the benefits of Wall Pilates and maintain an active and healthy lifestyle for years to come.